# Osteoporosis Diet Guide

## A 4-Step Bone-Building Plan Beyond Calcium (With Sample Meal Plans and Recipes)



mf

# Disclaimer

This guide is provided for informational and educational purposes only and should not be interpreted as medical, nutritional, or professional advice. The author is not a licensed physician, nurse, dietitian, or mental health provider. Reading this guide does not establish a patient–provider relationship of any kind.

Always seek the guidance of a qualified healthcare professional before starting, changing, or discontinuing any supplement, diet, or lifestyle program. If you are pregnant, breastfeeding, managing a chronic medical condition, or taking prescription medications, consult your physician or pharmacist before considering any product mentioned in this guide.

The author and publisher make no representations or warranties regarding accuracy, applicability, fitness, or completeness of the information contained herein. While every effort has been made to ensure scientific accuracy and currency, medical knowledge and research evolve continually. Readers are responsible for verifying information and making decisions in consultation with licensed professionals.

Use of this guide and any information contained within it is at your own risk. The author and publisher disclaim all liability

# Table of Contents

# Introduction

Osteoporosis is a progressive condition in which bones lose density and strength, increasing the risk of fractures even with minor falls or everyday stresses. Although many people recognize that calcium supports healthy bones, persistent misconceptions and dietary gaps undermine efforts to maintain optimal bone density. Common pitfalls such as over-reliance on a single nutrient or misinterpreting which foods genuinely support skeletal health often lead individuals to overlook critical elements of a comprehensive osteoporosis diet.

The global prevalence of osteoporosis is climbing as populations age, but this is not an unavoidable outcome of getting older. A significant number of cases go undiagnosed until a fracture occurs, resulting in substantial long-term health consequences such as impaired mobility and reduced independence. Suboptimal nutritional strategies further exacerbate bone loss, underscoring the urgent need for accurate, practical dietary guidance. Simply put, what you eat (and fail to eat) can be pivotal in either slowing down or accelerating the progression of osteoporosis.

This guide was created to provide you with practical and actionable knowledge to build and maintain stronger bones through food. It is specifically focused on dietary approaches, with a 4-step bone-building plan that moves beyond the outdated "just take calcium" mindset. Instead, it helps you assemble a nutrient-rich pattern of eating that targets the full spectrum of bone health needs using real food, smart meal planning, and science-backed guidelines.

Pharmaceutical treatments, exercise regimens, non-nutritional supplements, and genetic or secondary medical causes of osteoporosis are outside the scope of this guide. Here, the emphasis is on building a food-based defense for your bones demystifying the core dietary factors from protein and key vitamins and minerals to food preparation and meal composition.

Throughout the guide, you'll find:

- A streamlined overview of osteoporosis: what it is, how it progresses, and why nutrition matters in both prevention and ongoing care.
- The core principles of an osteoporosis-supportive diet, including insights into which nutrients matter most, how they interact, and how to maximize their absorption.
- A clear, four-step bone-building implementation system

Every section provides you with ready-to-use food selection checklists, sample meal plans, and complete recipes crafted for the osteoporosis diet. Real-world tips help troubleshoot common obstacles such as finding non-dairy calcium options or adjusting for dietary restrictions and are designed to fit daily routines and real budgets.

Tackling osteoporosis through diet may seem daunting, especially given the competing and sometimes confusing nutrition advice available. This guide cuts through the noise by focusing solely on the evidence-based, food-first methods that protect against bone loss, enhance nutrient intake, and fit into everyday life. By the end of this guide, you'll have a proven dietary framework clear, actionable, and adaptable to fortify your bones for the long run.

# Brief Overview of Osteoporosis (Fundamentals)

Osteoporosis is a chronic condition characterized by a reduction in bone mass and a deterioration of bone tissue strength. This invisible weakening leaves bones porous, fragile, and at an increased risk for fractures from minimal trauma. Though commonly associated with aging populations, osteoporosis often develops silently over decades, with no obvious symptoms until a break occurs. Understanding osteoporosis begins with clarifying what defines the disease, how it unfolds over time, and how it is clinically detected and, crucially, how diet and lifestyle shape both risk and progression.

## Osteoporosis Definition, Progression, and Clinical Diagnosis Framework

Osteoporosis is formally defined as a systemic skeletal disorder marked by compromised bone strength, predisposing individuals to an increased risk of fracture. Bone strength primarily reflects two critical components: bone density (the amount of mineral matter in bone) and bone quality (the architecture, turnover rate, and microdamage accumulation). While healthy bones constantly undergo a cycle of breakdown and rebuilding, osteoporosis tips the balance so that bone loss outpaces formation, resulting in bones that are thinner and structurally weaker.

The progression of osteoporosis moves in several distinctive phases. Peak bone mass is typically achieved in early adulthood, after which a gradual decline begins. This decline can accelerate dramatically particularly in women after menopause due to hormonal shifts that hasten bone resorption. In the absence of effective dietary and lifestyle interventions, this gradual depletion silently increases the risk of fracture, with the hip, spine, and wrist being especially vulnerable.

Osteoporosis is most commonly diagnosed using bone mineral density (BMD) measurements, usually assessed via dual-energy X-ray absorptiometry (DXA). A T-score of -2.5 or lower on a DXA scan qualifies as diagnostic for osteoporosis, while a T-score between -1.0 and -2.5 is classified as osteopenia (low bone mass, but not yet osteoporosis). Other clinical markers, such as a history of fragility fractures or radiographic evidence of vertebral compression, may also inform diagnosis and management pathways.

## Practical Risk Assessment Table: Key Risk Factors and Modifiable Triggers

While age and sex are non-modifiable risk factors, many other elements contributing to osteoporosis can be influenced most importantly, through diet and lifestyle choices. Below is a practical risk assessment table that highlights major contributors and modifiable triggers, with a focus on those actionable through nutrition and daily routines.

Table 1: Practical Osteoporosis Risk Assessment Table

| Risk Factor | Modifiable? | Nutritional Implication |
|---|---|---|
| Advancing age | No | Greater need for bone-supportive nutrients as absorption declines and hormonal changes occur |
| Female sex (post-menopause) | No | Estrogen loss increases bone loss; emphasize calcium, vitamin D, and overall bone nutrition |
| Family history of osteoporosis | No | Requires increased awareness and consistent bone-supportive dietary habits |
| Low dietary calcium intake | Yes | Weakens bone mineralization; increasing calcium-rich foods supports bone strength |
| Vitamin D deficiency | Yes | Reduces calcium absorption and bone formation; ensure adequate sunlight and dietary sources |
| Low protein intake | Yes | Limits bone matrix development; sufficient protein supports bone density maintenance |
| High sodium and processed food intake | Yes | Increases urinary calcium loss; reducing intake helps preserve bone mineral balance |

| Excess alcohol or caffeine intake | Yes | Overconsumption can interfere with bone formation and nutrient retention |
|---|---|---|
| Sedentary lifestyle | Yes | Lowers bone stimulation and often correlates with poorer diet quality |

Some risk factors, such as certain medications or chronic illnesses, are medically driven; however, the above table emphasizes those readily addressed by dietary intervention. The modifiable factors—low calcium, vitamin D, suboptimal protein, and excessive sodium feature prominently in the bone-building dietary plan outlined throughout this guide.

## Diagram of Bone Remodeling and Nutrient Roles

Bone is a dynamic tissue, maintained through a lifelong balance between two primary processes: formation (anabolic, performed by cells called osteoblasts) and breakdown (catabolic, managed by osteoclasts). Understanding bone remodeling is central to grasping how diet directly affects bone health.

### Diagram Description for In-Text Reference

At the center, imagine a cycle: Bone resorption (breakdown) by osteoclasts on one side, and bone formation by osteoblasts on the opposite. Key nutrients are mapped to their function along this cycle:

- Calcium and vitamin D are essential for new bone formation and mineralization.
- Magnesium supports bone structure and the activity of cells involved in bone formation.
- Vitamin K2 directs calcium into bone and out of blood vessels.
- Protein provides the fundamental matrix or scaffold for mineral deposition.
- Trace minerals, such as zinc, play a role in enzyme activity driving bone growth.

Excessive sodium, sugar, or alcohol is flagged as shifting the balance toward breakdown.]

**Specific Manifestations: Symptom and Screening Criteria Table**

Osteoporosis is widely known as a "silent disease," developing without prominent symptoms until a fracture occurs. However, some subtle manifestations may appear as bones weaken. Early recognition leads to timely screening and intervention.

Table 2: Symptom and Screening Criteria Table

| Manifestation | Screening or Diagnostic Indicator |
|---|---|
| Height loss or stooped posture | Measured reduction of 2cm+ in adult height or kyphosis |
| Sudden, unexplained back pain | Compression fractures evaluated by spinal X-rays or MRI |
| History of low-impact (fragility) fracture | Prompt BMD testing (DXA scan) and evaluation for osteoporosis |

| Family history of osteoporosis/ fractures | Clinical risk evaluation, may prompt earlier screening |
|---|---|
| Brittle or thinning nails | Nonspecific, but may be a dietary or metabolic signal |
| DEXA T-score below -2.5 | Diagnostic threshold for osteoporosis by World Health Organization criteria |
| Laboratory evidence of vitamin D deficiency or poor calcium status | Triggers nutritional assessment |

Since symptoms are often subtle, structured screening remains essential. Adults over 50, particularly women post-menopause or anyone with a family history of osteoporosis or prior low-trauma fracture, are candidates for periodic BMD testing.

## Hierarchical Taxonomy of Osteoporosis Types and Nutritional Implications

Not all osteoporosis develops for the same reasons or carries identical dietary management needs. The condition can be classified into several types, each with distinct nutritional implications.

**Hierarchical Taxonomy of Osteoporosis**

1. **Primary Osteoporosis**

    - Type I (Postmenopausal Osteoporosis):

      Predominantly affects women within 5-10 years after menopause due to estrogen deficiency, which accelerates bone turnover. Nutritionally, there is an urgent need to emphasize both calcium and vitamin D, but also to assure adequate protein and micronutrient intake to counter increased bone resorption.

- Type II (Age-Related or Senile Osteoporosis):

  Occurs in both men and women after age 70, associated with cumulative bone loss rather than hormonal shifts alone. Calcium absorption declines, so maximizing bioavailable calcium from various sources and ensuring diverse micronutrient intake (including magnesium and vitamin K2) becomes especially important.

2. **Secondary Osteoporosis**

   Linked to chronic medical conditions or medications (e.g., corticosteroids, anticonvulsants). While this guide does not address medication or disease management, it is important to stress that, in these types, nutritional therapy remains vital; particular attention should be paid to counteracting any nutrient loss or malabsorption due to medications or comorbidities.

**Nutritional Implications by Osteoporosis Type:**

- Postmenopausal women may need augmented nutrient intake as hormonal changes diminish bone protection.
- Older adults often require strategies to optimize nutrient absorption, focusing not only on calcium and vitamin D but also on a broader spectrum of micronutrients and high-quality protein.
- Secondary osteoporosis may demand targeted nutrient support to offset drug-nutrient interactions and maintain bone strength despite underlying disease.

This foundational understanding of osteoporosis lays the groundwork for the next steps in building an effective, comprehensive dietary strategy. Knowing how osteoporosis develops, how it is diagnosed, and which risk factors are responsive to nutritional choices empowers you to take a proactive role in bone health management.

The upcoming chapters will move beyond definitions and risk tables and provide you with a hands-on, stepwise approach to fortify your bones addressing not only calcium, but protein, vitamins, minerals, and the critical avoidance of bone-depleting additives. Practical food patterns, preparation guides, and real recipes will help turn these essentials into action for lifelong skeletal strength.

# Beyond Calcium—Core Principles of the Osteoporosis Diet (Fundamentals)

For decades, calcium has stood at the center of osteoporosis prevention and bone health conversations. While calcium is undoubtedly crucial for strong bones, focusing on this single nutrient leaves room for significant nutritional gaps that can undermine your progress. Modern osteoporosis nutrition recognizes that a comprehensive, multi-nutrient approach, one that considers how various vitamins, minerals, and even macronutrients interact is essential to building and preserving healthy bones for life. This chapter lays out the foundational knowledge you'll need to transform your meals into powerful allies in the fight against bone loss and fracture risk.

## Essential Bone-Protective Nutrients: The Foundation for Bone Health

The skeletal system relies on a complex array of nutrients beyond calcium. Each plays a unique role in building, maintaining, and defending bone tissue, and deficiencies sometimes even in the face of adequate calcium can compromise the strength and structure of your bones. The most important bone-protective nutrients include:

***Calcium*** is deposited in the collagen-rich framework of bone, providing the density measured in bone mineral tests. However, without sufficient vitamin D, much of your dietary calcium passes through the digestive system unused. Vitamin D, synthesized in the skin under sunlight or consumed in vitamin D-rich foods, enables calcium absorption and helps suppress excessive bone breakdown.

***Magnesium*** supports the transformation of vitamin D to its active blood form and stabilizes the bone's physical structure. Even moderate magnesium deficiency is linked to less robust bone and potentially to a higher risk of osteoporosis over time.

***Vitamin K2***'s role is to activate osteocalcin, a protein that binds calcium into the bone structure, and also to reduce the risk of calcium building up in blood vessels, a process associated with advanced bone loss and arterial problems.

***Protein*** serves as the sturdy "steel rebar" in bone's "concrete". It forms the collagenous framework into which minerals are deposited and supports ongoing repair processes. Older adults, in particular, can experience accelerated bone loss if protein intake is too low.

***Zinc, copper, manganese, and selenium*** each enable enzymatic reactions vital for bone production, antioxidant protection against bone cell damage, and connective tissue formation. While only needed in trace amounts, long-term shortfalls can erode bone strength.

## Absorption Rules and Interactive Effects: Nutrient Synergy and Antagonism

Not only is it important to get enough of each nutrient, but it is equally critical to understand how nutrients influence each other's absorption and physiological action. Some nutrients support each other's functions (synergy), while others can limit or even block absorption (antagonism). The illustration below acts as a mental "Nutrient Interaction Map" for optimizing your dietary patterns.

**Synergistic Nutrient Interactions:**

- ***Vitamin D and calcium***: Vitamin D increases intestinal uptake of calcium and helps deposit it into bone.
- ***Magnesium and vitamin D***: Magnesium is necessary to activate vitamin D, making vitamin D supplementation less effective if magnesium is chronically low.
- ***Vitamin K2 and calcium***: Vitamin K2 channels absorb calcium into bone tissue rather than allowing it to deposit in soft tissues.

- ***Protein and calcium***: Moderate, balanced protein intake aids in calcium retention in the skeleton, supporting a more robust bone framework.

**Antagonistic Nutrient Interactions:**

- ***Excess sodium and calcium***: Diets high in salt increase urinary calcium loss, depleting bone reserves.
- ***High phosphorus (especially from processed foods) and calcium***: Excessive phosphorus can disrupt the balance with calcium, leading to bone demineralization if not offset by sufficient calcium intake.
- ***Oxalates (in certain greens, like spinach) and calcium***: Oxalate-rich foods can bind dietary calcium in the gut, lowering its absorption. Vary calcium sources for better absorption.
- ***Excessive caffeine and calcium***: Excess caffeine intake can slightly reduce calcium absorption and boost its excretion.

Applying these principles, prioritize a diet that provides a broad spectrum of these nutrients across the day, limiting factors (such as high sodium, soft drinks, and processed foods) that interfere with mineral balance.

## Guidelines for Optimizing Bioavailability of Bone-Building Nutrients from Whole Foods

Bioavailability refers to the degree to which a nutrient is absorbed and utilized by the body. Maximizing the bioavailability of bone-nourishing nutrients means focusing on their most accessible forms and preparing foods to unlock their full value:

1. ***Diversify Food Sources***: Different foods offer varying forms and ratios of minerals and vitamins. Leafy greens (like kale or bok choy) provide bioavailable calcium with less oxalate than spinach. Fatty fish and fortified dairy deliver vitamin D, while nuts and legumes are rich in magnesium.
2. ***Pair Foods for Synergy***: Serve vitamin D-rich foods (e.g., salmon) with calcium-containing items (e.g., fortified plant milk or low-oxalate greens) to enhance calcium absorption. Include healthy fats (from avocado, olive oil, or nuts) to increase vitamin D and K2 absorption.
3. ***Use Cooking Techniques to Reduce Antagonists***: Soaking or sprouting beans, seeds, and grains lowers phytate content, which otherwise can bind minerals and hinder their absorption. Lightly steaming greens reduces oxalate, improving calcium availability.
4. ***Avoid Large Doses of Competing Minerals Simultaneously***: Large amounts of supplemental zinc,

calcium, or iron can block each other's absorption. Spread intake throughout the day for best results.

5. ***Focus on Moderate Sodium Intake***: Prepare meals with fresh ingredients and light seasoning, limiting processed foods to reduce sodium-driven urinary calcium loss.

Select Naturally Fortified and Fermented Foods: Some options, such as certain yogurts and cheeses, are natural sources of vitamin K2. Consuming eggs and fermented foods occasionally can also help raise K2 levels.

Incorporating these strategies can significantly improve the absorption of bone-supporting nutrients from whole foods. Thoughtful food choices and preparation methods help ensure that essential vitamins and minerals are available to support bone health. Small adjustments in your daily eating habits can make a meaningful difference over time.

## Recipe Modification Framework for Enhancing Nutrient Density

Upgrading everyday meals for osteoporosis support does not require drastic changes it's about smart substitutions, additions, and tweaks that layer in bone-protective nutrients:

- ***Replace white rice, pasta, or bread with*** whole grain versions to boost magnesium, zinc, and fiber.

- ***Add a handful of chopped nuts or seeds*** (such as almonds or sesame) to salads, breakfast bowls, or yogurt for a magnesium and protein lift.
- ***Swap iceberg lettuce with dark, leafy greens*** like kale, collard greens, or arugula in salads for dramatically higher calcium and vitamin K content.
- ***Enrich soups, stews, and casseroles*** with beans or lentils, offering both protein and trace minerals.
- ***Use small fish with edible bones*** (like sardines) or tofu prepared with calcium sulfate to raise total calcium.
- ***Enhance omelets, stir-fries, or grain bowls*** with mushrooms and fortified plant-based milks for a natural vitamin D boost.
- ***Opt for homemade dressings*** with olive oil and apple cider vinegar to assist fat-soluble vitamin absorption without added sodium.
- ***Limit added sugars***, which not only lower the overall nutrient density but can also interfere with calcium uptake over time.

When following recipes, scan ingredient lists and preparation techniques for nutrient opportunities: Can you add seeds or nuts, swap a grain, slip in baby spinach, or include a fermented food alongside the main dish? Consider blending in cooked white beans for creamy texture and bonus protein/minerals in soups or dips.

### Checklist for Identifying Hidden Nutritional Pitfalls in Common Diets

Even diets that appear healthy on the surface can harbor hidden risks for bone health if not carefully assessed. Use this checklist to audit your current eating patterns and meal choices:

- ☐ Are you consuming an abundance of processed or convenience foods that are high in sodium, which increases calcium excretion?
- ☐ Does your daily fluid intake rely heavily on soft drinks or sweetened beverages, which can be high in phosphates that throw off the calcium/phosphorus balance?
- ☐ Is most of your calcium coming from high-oxalate plants (spinach, beet greens) that significantly reduce its absorption, without variety from lower-oxalate sources?
- ☐ Do you skip or marginalize protein at meals, especially at breakfast or lunch? Consistently low protein can speed up bone loss as you age.
- ☐ Are plant-based meals characterized by lots of grains and beans but little attention to vitamin B12 and D sources, which are often lacking in unfortified diets?
- ☐ Are you over-relying on calcium-fortified snack bars or beverages, which often come with added sugars and

sodium but lack the full spectrum of bone-building nutrients?

- ☐ Do you eat little/no fermented foods or healthy fats, thereby missing natural sources of vitamin K2 and support for fat-soluble vitamin absorption?
- ☐ Are caffeinated drinks or alcohol consumed in excess, crowding out bone-supportive hydration and increasing mineral losses?
- ☐ Do you routinely avoid or severely limit all dairy and fortified plant alternatives without a thoughtful plan for adequate calcium, D, and protein?

Honest answers to these questions may uncover gaps or excesses that require targeted adjustments. The osteoporosis diet is not about just adding calcium success depends on a thoughtful integration of the full range of nutrients while avoiding bone-depleting elements.

To build and preserve bone strength, a truly effective osteoporosis diet must move well past singling out calcium. The pattern that best supports your skeleton is built on deliberate inclusion of a range of vitamins, minerals, high-quality proteins, and careful attention to how foods are prepared and combined. By understanding the essential nutrients involved, respecting nutrient interactions, choosing preparation methods that improve absorption, modifying recipes for maximum nutrient density, and keeping watch for subtle dietary pitfalls, your meals can work harder for your bones every single day.

Remember, successful diet strategies are not one-dimensional. When every meal is viewed as an opportunity to boost not just calcium, but D, K2, magnesium, protein, and the supportive cast of trace elements, you lay a stronger foundation for lifelong skeletal health.

# Step 1 of the Bone-Building Plan—Optimizing Protein Intake (Application)

**Protein's Critical Role in the Osteoporosis Diet**

Optimizing protein intake represents a foundational first step in any osteoporosis nutrition plan. Protein is not simply an accessory to minerals like calcium, it is actively involved in building, repairing, and maintaining the living matrix that forms the core structure of your bones. This chapter breaks down protein's unique roles in skeletal health, how to calculate your individual needs, and how to fold the best protein sources into a bone-protective meal pattern.

## Protein and Bone Matrix Formation

Bones are not static or inert; they are constantly being remodeled; old bone breaks down and is replaced by newly formed bone tissue. At the heart of this dynamic process is a collagen-based matrix. Protein, particularly certain amino acids, supplies the fundamental building blocks of this collagen network. Without enough protein, the bone matrix becomes thin and brittle, unable to properly bind the minerals (such as calcium, magnesium, and phosphate) that give bone its density and strength.

Beyond structural support, protein also affects hormones and signaling molecules that regulate bone turnover rate. Adequate protein intake is correlated with reduced risk of low bone mass, falls, and subsequent fractures, especially in older adults and those already experiencing bone loss. Meeting the right protein targets helps preserve muscle strength as well as a crucial factor for mobility and reducing fall risk, both significant contributors to fracture rates in osteoporosis.

**Daily Protein Requirement Calculation Tool**

To put these principles into practice, you need a personal target for daily protein intake. The most widely accepted range for adults seeking to support optimal bone health is between 1.0 and 1.2 grams of protein per kilogram (kg) of body weight per day. This is slightly higher than the recommended dietary allowance for the general population, reflecting the increased importance of protein for older adults and those with, or at risk for, osteoporosis.

To calculate your daily protein requirement:

1. Find your weight in kilograms. (To convert from pounds, divide weight in pounds by 2.2.)
2. Multiply your weight in kilograms by 1.0–1.2.

Example: If you weigh 150 pounds (68 kg), your target range is 68–82 grams per day (68 kg × 1.0 and 68 kg × 1.2).

Factors that may increase protein needs include advanced age, recent fracture, or concurrent muscle loss. If you are underweight, have a history of hip or vertebral fracture, or are recovering from surgery or illness, target the higher end of this range. Always consult your healthcare provider to tailor dietary targets to your specific situation.

## Protein Source Table: Complete and Incomplete Proteins for Osteoporosis Support

Not all protein is created equal, particularly when it comes to supporting strong bones. Proteins from food are made up of amino acids. "Complete proteins" contain all nine essential amino acids your body cannot make, while "incomplete proteins" are missing one or more of these building blocks.

To optimize both total intake and amino acid profile, focus on a mix of both complete and complementary incomplete protein sources:

Table 3: Protein Source Table

| Complete Proteins (all essential amino acids) | Incomplete Proteins (combine for full amino acid coverage) |
|---|---|
| Eggs | Beans, lentils, chickpeas |
| Dairy products (milk, yogurt, cheese) | |
| Poultry (chicken, turkey) | Nuts and seeds (almonds, sunflower seeds, pumpkin seeds) |
| Fish and seafood (salmon, sardines, trout) | |
| Lean red meat | Whole grains (brown rice, barley, oats, whole wheat) |
| Soy foods (tofu, tempeh, edamame, soy milk) | |
| Quinoa | Vegetables (broccoli, spinach, peas) |
| Buckwheat | |

Pairing different incomplete protein sources (such as beans and rice, or peanut butter and whole wheat bread) over the course of the day ensures your body receives all the essential amino acids required for bone matrix formation.

## Decision Rules for Balancing Animal and Plant-Based Protein in Meal Construction

Both animal and plant proteins offer advantages for bone health, but they differ in amino acid completeness, bioavailability, and accompanying nutrients. Here are practical guidelines for balancing these sources:

1. ***Prioritize Variety***: Aim to include both animal and plant-based proteins over the week. This provides a broader nutrient spectrum: animal sources boost

vitamin B12, bioavailable calcium (if using dairy), and easily absorbed amino acids, while plant sources deliver fiber, phytochemicals, magnesium, and potassium.

2. ***Maximize Quality Within Preferences***: If you eat animal products, low-fat dairy, eggs, chicken, fish, and small servings of lean red meat supply complete protein efficiently. For plant-based diets, pay special attention to food pairing (grains and legumes) to maximize essential amino acid intake.
3. ***Watch Portion Size and Saturated Fat***: For animal proteins, opt for lean cuts and limit processed meats, which contain added sodium and preservatives. For plant-based sources, watch portion sizes for higher-calorie options like nuts and seeds, but appreciate their mineral and healthy fat content.
4. ***Include Calcium-Rich Options***: For every major protein source, consider its contribution to your daily calcium goal choose dairy, calcium-set tofu, or canned fish with bones for a dual nutrient benefit.
5. ***Limit Bone-Depleting Additives***: Avoid or minimize protein sources high in sodium, such as processed cheeses, deli meats, and salted nuts, as excess sodium promotes urinary calcium loss.

Applying these decision rules helps ensure each meal and snack not only meets protein targets but also supports your bone health holistically.

## Sample Substitution Guidelines for Common Low-Protein Meals

Many traditional meals and snacks are low in protein, missing a key opportunity for bone building. Simple substitutions and upgrades transform meals into more effective partners in your osteoporosis diet strategy:

**Breakfast:**

- Instead of white toast with jam, try whole grain toast smeared with nut butter or topped with scrambled eggs.
- Swap fruit-only smoothies for versions blended with Greek yogurt or a scoop of plant-based protein powder.
- Replace refined breakfast cereals with overnight oats, folded in chia seeds or finely chopped nuts.

**Lunch:**

- Instead of a plain green salad, add grilled chicken, canned salmon (with bones), tofu cubes, or a scoop of beans, plus seeds for crunch.
- Upgrade vegetable soup by mixing in lentils or shredded turkey.

**Snacks:**

- Swap crackers for cottage cheese with pineapple, or hummus with raw veggie sticks.

- Replace sweet granola bars with hard-boiled eggs, a small portion of roasted chickpeas, or a cheese stick paired with whole grain crackers.

**Dinner:**

- Instead of white pasta with tomato sauce, opt for lentil or chickpea-based pasta, or add sautéed ground turkey, sardines, or tempeh to your sauce.
- If using stir-fry, double the protein by including both tofu and a sprinkle of sesame seeds or peanuts.

These substitutions not only raise protein content but also boost supporting minerals and vitamins vital for bone integrity.

## Weekly Protein Intake Tracking Sheet for Diet Adherence

Maintaining consistent protein intake is easier when you track your progress. Use this simple weekly tracker to monitor daily totals and spot patterns that may need adjusting:

**Weekly Protein Intake Tracking Sheet**

- Create a table with columns for each day (Monday through Sunday).
- Record the total grams of protein consumed at the end of each day.

- Use a notes column to log which meals fell short and which exceeded your target.

Table 3: Example Tracking Table

| Day | Total Protein (g) | Notes |
|---|---|---|
| Monday | 74 | Lunch low—add beans |
| Tuesday | 82 | On target |
| Wednesday | 65 | Low at breakfast |
| Thursday | 89 | High—chose double protein |
| Friday | 77 | On target |
| Saturday | 70 | Replace afternoon snack |
| Sunday | 80 | Good variety |

Regularly reviewing this sheet helps you identify trends, maintain accountability, and ensure you meet intake targets needed for bone protection and repair.

**Practical Insights and Action Steps**

1. Don't skip protein at breakfast or lunch—distribute intake across all main meals and snacks, rather than saving most for the evening.
2. Include at least one full serving (7–14g for snacks, 20–30g for main meals) of high-quality protein.
3. When in doubt, "layer up" protein in your meals: Add seeds to yogurt, beans to soups, or eggs to stir-fries.
4. If relying heavily on plant-based proteins, check that grains and legumes are represented daily.
5. Choose minimally processed options—homemade or low-sodium foods whenever possible.

## Troubleshooting Common Pitfalls

Missing protein at breakfast is a leading reason for falling short on daily intake. If you are often rushed, consider prepping boiled eggs, overnight protein oats, or nut butter sandwiches in advance. For those with sensitive digestive systems, space protein intake throughout the day and favor gentle sources, like baked fish, soft tofu, or milder legumes.

If your total daily calories are low due to appetite loss (common with age or illness), focus on more concentrated protein sources such as Greek yogurt, cottage cheese, nut butters, small portions of high-protein smoothies rather than filling up on bulkier foods with less protein per bite.

Optimizing protein intake forms the backbone, quite literally, of an effective osteoporosis diet. By understanding the critical functions of protein in bone formation and fracture prevention, calculating your ideal daily goal, and consciously selecting nutrient-dense protein sources (both animal and plant-based), you lay a firm foundation for the rest of your bone-building plan. Use the protein source table, substitution guidelines, and weekly tracking tools provided to ensure your diet delivers consistent support for lifelong skeletal health.

# Step 2 of the Bone-Building Plan—Ensuring Adequate Vitamins and Trace Nutrients (Application)

Moving beyond optimizing protein intake, the second step in a comprehensive osteoporosis diet plan is ensuring you obtain a steady and adequate supply of crucial vitamins and trace minerals. While calcium is often in the spotlight, several other micronutrients, especially vitamin D, vitamin K2, magnesium, and zinc work in concert to fortify bone structure, regulate bone metabolism, and reduce the risk of fractures. This chapter explores practical strategies for identifying and incorporating these bone-building micronutrients, optimizing their absorption, and navigating common barriers that can hinder your progress.

## Selection Grid for Vitamin D, Vitamin K2, Magnesium, and Zinc-Rich Whole Foods

Assembling an osteoporosis-friendly menu requires recognition of dietary sources that deliver more than just calcium. Use the following food selection grid for day-to-day guidance, focusing on real, minimally processed foods that provide optimal concentrations of these vital nutrients:

**Vitamin D**

- Fatty fish (salmon, mackerel, sardines, trout)
- Cod liver oil
- Fortified dairy (milk, yogurt), and plant milks (soy, almond, oat, when labeled)
- Egg yolks
- Fortified cereals

**Vitamin K2**

- Natto (fermented soybeans)
- Aged cheeses (Gouda, Edam, Jarlsberg)
- Kefir and other fermented dairy products
- Pasture-raised eggs
- Chicken thighs and drumsticks, especially from free-range sources

**Magnesium**

- Pumpkin seeds, chia seeds, sunflower seeds
- Almonds, cashews, peanuts
- Spinach, Swiss chard, beet greens
- Black beans, lentils, chickpeas
- Whole grains (quinoa, brown rice, oats)

**Zinc**

- Oysters, crab, lobster
- Lean beef, pork, and chicken (especially dark meat)
- Pumpkin seeds, sesame seeds
- Chickpeas, lentils, kidney beans
- Fortified whole grain cereals

Strive to mix a variety of these foods across your weekly meal plan to evenly distribute your intake, paying special attention to pairing animal and plant sources for dietary variety and synergy.

## Vitamin D Synthesis Factors: Stepwise Optimization Checklist

Vitamin D is unique among bone-supportive nutrients because your body can synthesize it with adequate sunlight exposure. However, a multitude of factors can impact your vitamin D status. Follow this stepwise checklist to maximize your vitamin D levels through both lifestyle and dietary choices:

1. **Evaluate Sun Exposure:**
    - Aim for 10–30 minutes of midday sun exposure on arms and legs, several times per week. Timing and skin area exposed matter.

- Take note of latitude, season, skin pigmentation, age, and sunscreen use, all of which can reduce vitamin D production.

2. **Incorporate Dietary Sources:**
   - Integrate vitamin D-rich foods (see grid above) regularly, especially if sun exposure is limited.
   - Read labels; many non-dairy milks and breakfast cereals are fortified, but always verify fortification amounts.

3. **Facilitate Absorption:**
   - Pair vitamin D foods with healthy fats (olive oil, avocados, nuts) to enhance absorption, as vitamin D is fat-soluble.
   - Ensure a baseline of adequate digestive health; malabsorption syndromes or certain gut surgeries can impair vitamin D uptake.

4. **Monitor and Adjust:**
   - Consider annual vitamin D blood level checks, especially if you are older, have darker skin, are overweight, or follow a vegan diet.
   - Work with your healthcare provider if your levels fall short; food may not always be sufficient to meet needs in all individuals.

By addressing each point in this checklist, you reduce the risk of vitamin D deficiency, which is strongly associated with increased bone turnover and fragility.

### Common Obstacles to Micronutrient Sufficiency and Adjustment Rules

Despite careful meal planning, a number of obstacles can compromise micronutrient sufficiency:

- ***Low Dietary Intake***: Restrictive or highly selective diets (those limiting dairy, animal products, or grains) may chronically undersupply one or more bone-relevant nutrients.
- ***Poor Absorption***: Gastrointestinal issues (such as celiac or Crohn's disease), certain medications (proton pump inhibitors, some antacids), or age-associated digestive changes may hamper nutrient uptake.
- ***Drug-Nutrient Interactions***: Some medications can increase urinary loss or decrease absorption of magnesium and zinc.
- ***Lifestyle Factors***: Excessive alcohol usage, high-phytate/oxalate intake (from large amounts of unsoaked beans, raw spinach), and chronic stress can diminish micronutrient status.

### Adjustment Rules:

- If any barrier to absorption or intake exists, prioritize higher-density sources (e.g., natto for vitamin K2, pumpkin seeds for magnesium and zinc, fortified foods for vitamin D).

- Cook or lightly steam high-oxalate or high-phytate foods to improve magnesium and zinc absorption.
- Include fermented foods (yogurt, kefir, sauerkraut) to increase vitamin K2 and enhance gut environment for nutrient uptake.
- If supplementing, always coordinate with a healthcare professional to prevent overcompensation, toxicity, or adverse interactions.
- Regular nutritional screening: If you have chronic digestive or malabsorption issues, annual lab assessments for vitamin D, magnesium, and zinc are recommended.

## Absorption Boundaries and Timing Tactics for Improving Nutrient Uptake

Absorption is as critical as intake—nutrients must transit the digestive system to be useful for bone health. Consider these boundary conditions and timing tactics:

### Vitamin D:

Fat-soluble, so best absorbed with meals containing some fat. Spreading intake and pairing with lunch or dinner optimizes absorption.

**Vitamin K2:**

Also fat-soluble; serve K2-rich foods (cheese, eggs) alongside olive oil-based dressings or avocado.

**Magnesium:**

- High fiber and phytate intakes can inhibit absorption. Soak or cook legumes and grains to lower blocking agents.
- Split large doses: If consuming magnesium-rich foods or supplements, divide into two servings—morning and evening—to reduce gastrointestinal upset and maximize uptake.

**Zinc:**

- Competes with iron and calcium for absorption. Avoid taking zinc-rich meals with high-dose calcium or iron supplements at the same time.
- Try combining plant-based zinc foods with citrus or vitamin C-rich foods (lemon juice on lentil salad, tomatoes in bean stews) to boost bioavailability.

**General Tips:**

- Spread micronutrient-rich foods throughout the day rather than piling into a single meal.
- Avoid reliance on "superfoods"—diversity and consistent intake trump any one ingredient.

Optimizing nutrient absorption involves more than simply choosing the right foods—it requires attention to timing, food combinations, and preparation methods. Small adjustments, like pairing fat-soluble vitamins with meals or spacing out mineral intake, can make a significant difference in bone health. Consistent, varied intake throughout the day ensures your body gets the most benefit from your diet.

## Table Ranking Daily Micronutrient Targets for Osteoporosis Prevention

The table below provides practical, research-aligned daily intake targets for the key micronutrients supporting bone health. These values are appropriate for most adults seeking to reduce the risk or progression of osteoporosis. Always consult with your healthcare provider for personal adjustments based on your clinical status, medication use, age, or coexisting health concerns.

Table 4: Daily Micronutrient Targets

| Micronutrient | Recommended Daily Intake (Adults) |
| --- | --- |
| Vitamin D | 600–800 IU (higher needs in older adults) |
| Vitamin K2 | 90–120 mcg |
| Magnesium | 310–420 mg |
| Zinc | 8–11 mg |

### Practical Application: Building Your Daily Plan

Applying these principles need not be complicated. Here's how to structure a typical bone-wise day:

***Breakfast***: Fortified oatmeal with pumpkin seeds and sliced almonds. Pair with a boiled egg and a glass of vitamin D-fortified orange juice.

***Lunch***: Lentil and spinach salad, sprinkled with sunflower seeds, dressed in olive oil and lemon. Include a serving of aged cheese or kefir.

***Snack***: Greek yogurt mixed with berries and a spoonful of chia seeds.

***Dinner***: Oven-baked salmon or sardines, with a side of sautéed Swiss chard and brown rice. Lightly steamed broccoli as a magnesium booster.

Throughout the week, swap ingredients for other items from the provided selection grid to prevent menu fatigue and maximize trace nutrient intake.

### Troubleshooting: When Targets Aren't Met

If analysis of your meal plan reveals repeated shortfalls in any micronutrient:

- Increase frequency of the highest-yield sources for that nutrient (e.g., commit to oily fish twice weekly for vitamin D, or natto several times for K2).
- Adjust snacks to include nuts, seeds, or yogurts tailored to your goals.

- For vegetarians or vegans, pay special attention to K2 (fermented foods), magnesium (leafy greens, beans), and zinc (soaked/sprouted legumes).

Remember, small consistent shifts—like switching from white to whole grain bread, or adding extra seeds to breakfast—aggregate into meaningful improvements.

# Step 3 of the Bone-Building Plan—Limiting Bone-Depleting Foods and Additives (Mechanisms)

A critical but frequently overlooked piece of a robust osteoporosis diet isn't just about what you add to your plate; it's also about what you avoid. Many common foods, additives, and even the way foods are processed can undermine efforts to maintain and rebuild healthy bone mass.

This chapter supplies a detailed blueprint for identifying and limiting bone-depleting foods and ingredients, demystifies how the acid-base balance of the diet impacts mineral status, gives you practical tools for decoding product labels, and provides an evidence-based approach to eliminating common culprits for stronger bones.

## List of High-Sodium, Excessive Caffeine, and Sugar-Containing Foods and Additives with Bone-Negative Impact Scores

Various foods and ingredients have an established bone-negative effect because they either increase the loss of calcium from the body, interfere with nutrient absorption, or otherwise alter bone metabolism. It's not only about obvious culprits like cola but also about a hidden network of additives in many packaged foods. Here's a targeted index of key categories that deserve your attention, ranked according to their documented negative impact on bone health:

### High-Sodium Foods

- ***Processed meats*** (bacon, ham, deli slices, sausage): Sodium content can reach over 1,000 mg per serving—far above optimal daily targets for those concerned about bone health.
- ***Canned soups and broths***: Often contain 700–900 mg sodium per cup.
- ***Snack foods*** (chips, flavored pretzels, crackers): Sodium levels can quietly accumulate with small servings.
- ***Fast food entrees and sandwiches***: Frequently exceed 1,500 mg sodium per meal.
- ***Store-bought sauces, condiments, and dressings***: Especially soy sauce, jarred pasta sauce, salad dressings, and pickles.

**Excessive-Caffeine Foods and Drinks**

- ***Brewed coffee***: Over 2–3 cups per day (about 250–300 mg caffeine) can increase urinary calcium loss.
- ***Energy drinks and shots***: With 80–200 mg caffeine per serving, often combined with sweeteners.
- ***Cola beverages***: Contain both caffeine and phosphoric acid—each linked to lower bone density.
- ***Certain teas***: Black and green tea have lower caffeine, but large amounts or concentrate can still pose risks.

**Sugar-Containing Foods and Additives**

- ***Sweetened soft drinks*** (especially cola): Sugar plus phosphoric acid is a problematic duo.
- ***Candy, pastries, muffins, and commercial cakes***: Often have high levels of both sugar and hidden sodium.
- ***Breakfast bars and granola***: Sometimes "masked" with claims of health but loaded with added sugars, syrups, and sodium.
- ***Flavored yogurts and puddings***: Sugar content can overshadow the benefits of the base dairy.
- ***Condensed milk, low-fat dairy desserts, and flavored milks***: Sugar can offset the bone-supporting benefits of their proteins and minerals.

These foods, when regularly consumed, tip the nutritional balance in favor of bone breakdown, and accumulate risk over time. While occasional small servings can fit into some meal plans, anyone managing osteoporosis should become proficient at recognizing and limiting their presence.

## Acid-Base Load Foods and Their Effect on Bone Mineral Balance: Acidic/Alkaline Food Impact

The "acid-base load" of your diet is the net effect it has on blood chemistry once foods are digested and metabolized. Diets high in acid-forming foods can, over many years, promote increased calcium loss as the body mobilizes alkaline minerals (like calcium and magnesium) from bone to buffer acids in the bloodstream. Conversely, diets that emphasize alkaline-forming foods lower this burden and may be bone protective.

Below is a simplified Acidic/Alkaline Food Impact to guide your daily choices:

**Acidic Foods (Increase Acid Load—Reduce or Moderate)**

- Processed meats (hot dogs, bacon, ham)
- Cheese (especially hard, highly salted varieties)
- White breads, refined pasta, white rice
- Most animal proteins (beef, pork, poultry—not to be excluded, but balance is key)
- Sugar-sweetened beverages (cola, flavored water, energy drinks)
- Most pastries, cookies, and sweet snacks

**Alkaline-Forming Foods (Reduce Acid Load—Promote)**

- Most fresh fruits (bananas, oranges, melons, berries, apples)
- Vegetables (especially leafy greens, broccoli, squash, zucchini, bell peppers)
- Legumes and beans (lentils, black beans, chickpeas)
- Nuts and seeds (almonds, chia, pumpkin; consume in balanced quantities for calorie control)
- Whole grains (quinoa, brown rice, buckwheat, millet)

***Balanced Diet Principle***: The goal is not to eliminate all acid-forming foods. Adequate protein from animal and plant sources is still essential for bone health. Focus instead on offsetting higher-protein meals with generous servings of alkalizing plant foods each day. For most, a 60–70% emphasis on alkaline-forming foods is a practical and beneficial target.

## Checklist for Reading Labels to Spot Hidden Bone-Depleting Ingredients

Many of the bone-depleting agents in foods are not obvious from front-of-package claims. Use this label-reading checklist when shopping for packaged, canned, or convenience foods:

1. **Scan the sodium line on Nutrition Facts:**

   Look for <140 mg per serving for "low sodium" and aim to keep daily sodium intake as close to

1,500–2,000 mg as possible, unless your healthcare provider gives you specific guidance.

2. **Locate added sugars in both grams and ingredients list:**
    - Choose products with <5g added sugar per serving where possible.
    - Watch for "hidden" sugars labeled as corn syrup, maltose, sucrose, fructose, dextrose, honey, agave, concentrated fruit juice.
3. **Identify caffeine sources:**

    On beverages, look for both "caffeine content" (if provided) or decode sources ("coffee concentrate," "guarana," "yerba mate," "black tea extract").

4. **Check for phosphate additives:**

    Ingredients like "sodium phosphate," "calcium phosphate," "phosphoric acid" are sometimes added to enhance texture or shelf life and can add to excess phosphorus intake, a consideration especially with cola drinks and many processed meats.

5. **Monitor "serving size" trickery:**

    Manufacturers may list nutrient values for unrealistically small servings. Multiply numbers by the typical consumption amount.

6. **Beware of "Reduced Fat" or "Low-Calorie" marketing:**

   Many such products add salt, sugar, or artificial sweeteners to boost flavor when fat is removed.

7. **Look for fortification and balance:**

   Fortified foods can supply nutrients helpful for bone, but always weigh the benefit of added vitamin D or calcium against a possibly high sodium or sugar load.

## Sample One-Week Elimination Experiment Protocol for Common Dietary Culprits

If you are unsure how your usual choices may be affecting your bone health, a one-week dietary elimination experiment can provide clarity and a jump-start for healthier habits. Follow this protocol for best results:

### Days 1–2: Audit Your Normal Diet

Write down everything you eat or drink, focusing on sodium, caffeine sources, sweetened products, and processed snacks or meals.

### Days 3–7: Eliminate or Drastically Limit Common Bone-Depleting Foods

- ***Avoid***: All processed meats, canned soups/broths, fast food, sweetened beverages, commercial baked goods, and highly salted packaged snacks.

- ***Limit***: Brewed coffee and caffeinated tea to $\leq 1$ cup/day, opt for water, herbal teas, or unsweetened plant milks.
- ***Replace***: Swap out white bread/pasta for 100% whole grains, increase fresh or steamed vegetables and fruits at every meal.
- ***Add***: Use herbs, spices, and lemon juice in place of salt; try natural nut butters, seeds, and unsweetened yogurts as snacks.
- ***Track***: At the close of each day, review your intake against the "avoid" and "add" lists.

**Optional**: Keep a log of how you feel, any changes in energy, digestion, fluid retention, and mood. While these may not directly measure bone health, many people notice improvements in overall well-being within just a few days of a lower-sodium, whole-food-rich eating pattern.

## Risk Guide to Popular Processed Food and Drink Categories

Given the sheer variety of processed foods and drinks, it can be tough to quickly judge their relative bone health risk. Use this simple risk matrix to guide decisions when considering store bought or restaurant foods:

**High-Risk (Limit or Avoid)**

- Salty packaged snacks: potato chips, cheese puffs, pretzel sticks, microwave popcorn with seasoning packs.
- Processed and cured meats: ham, bacon, sausage, hot dogs, beef jerky.
- Sweetened and/or caffeinated soft drinks: regular and diet colas, "energy" sodas, sweet iced teas.
- Flavored instant noodles and boxed meal kits: typically high in both sodium and phosphate additives.
- Bakery products: donuts, muffins, commercial cakes with frosting, prepacked cookies.

**Moderate-Risk (Use Sparingly or Modify)**

- Restaurant soups, salads with creamy/packaged dressings, sandwich spreads.
- Ready-to-eat breakfast cereals: particularly those with less fiber or added sugar.
- Flavored yogurts and "light" desserts: can be chosen with care (look for plain or unsweetened alternatives and add your own fruit).
- Spiced nut or seed mixes: even healthy nuts can be overly salted or sugared.

**Low-Risk (Typically Bone Neutral or Positive)**

- Plain, unsweetened yogurts (add fresh fruit for flavor).
- Fresh or frozen fruits and vegetables without sauces.

- Whole, unprocessed grains (brown rice, quinoa, steel-cut oats).
- Lean, unseasoned poultry or fish prepared at home.
- Raw or dry-roasted unsalted nuts and seeds.

Armed with this matrix, aim to build your regular meals and snacks from the low-risk options, using moderate-risk foods strategically and high-risk items only on rare occasions.

# Step 4 of the Bone-Building Plan—Creating a Whole-Food Meal Pattern (Systems)

A bone-supportive diet is not just a list of single nutrients or isolated "superfoods." The strength of any osteoporosis prevention or management strategy lies in creating a cohesive, whole-food meal pattern—a system that weaves together diversity, balance, and practical routines. Step 4 of the Bone-Building Plan integrates all previous nutritional pillars into actionable daily meal systems, ensuring a continuous, easy-to-follow approach that becomes a living habit rather than a sporadic checklist.

## Sample Weekly Meal Planning Template for Balanced Nutrient Coverage

A structured weekly meal plan helps you cover the full spectrum of nutrients needed to protect and rebuild bone. It also streamlines your grocery shopping and reduces the mental burden of daily decision-making. Below is a template for a standard week, emphasizing whole foods that maximize calcium, vitamin D, magnesium, protein, vitamin K2, and trace minerals:

- ***Breakfasts***: Prioritize calcium-rich or fortified dairy or plant alternatives with high-protein additions (e.g., Greek yogurt and berries; fortified soy milk with oatmeal and walnuts).
- ***Lunch***: Rotate leafy greens as salad bases, include a protein source (chickpeas, grilled chicken, canned salmon), and add a whole grain (quinoa, brown rice, buckwheat).
- ***Dinners***: Aim for half the plate as vegetables (at least one dark leafy green), a palm-sized source of protein, a serving of whole grain or starchy root, and a topping of nuts or seeds.
- ***Snacks***: Mix nuts or seeds with fresh fruit, vegetable sticks with hummus, cottage cheese with pineapple, or a hard-boiled egg with cherry tomatoes.

Table 5: Weekly Template (example layout)

| | **Monday** | **Tuesday** | **Wednesday** |
|---|---|---|---|
| **Breakfast** | Oatmeal w/ almonds + berries | Egg scramble + spinach | Greek yogurt + granola |
| **Lunch** | Lentil-spinach salad + feta | Turkey & kale wrap + apple | Chickpea, arugula & olive bowl |
| **Snack 1** | 1 orange | Walnuts | Banana |
| **Dinner** | Salmon, brown rice, broccoli | Tofu stir-fry, quinoa, cabbage | Grilled chicken, millet, chard |
| **Snack 2** | Yogurt | Pear | Cottage cheese |

**The guiding principle**: Each meal and snack intentionally features at least two bone-supporting food groups (dairy or fortified equivalents; greens, nuts/seeds, whole grains, seafood or legumes), spaced throughout the day for coverage and absorption.

## Food Group Prioritization Rules in a Meal Pattern Design Guide

Certain food groups have well-documented benefits in the osteoporosis diet. Following prioritization rules in meal design can ensure consistent daily intake of the most crucial nutrients:

1. **Dairy and Fortified Dairy Alternatives:**

   Feature at least 2 servings per day for optimal calcium and protein. These can include milk, yogurt, kefir, or fortified plant milks. For dairy-sensitive or vegan eaters, select calcium- and vitamin D-fortified soy, almond, or oat beverages, reading labels to confirm fortification.

2. **Leafy Greens:**

   Integrate a minimum of 1.5–2 cups daily, rotating between spinach, kale, bok choy, collards, and arugula. These contribute calcium, magnesium, vitamin K, and a spectrum of phytochemicals.

3. **Nuts and Seeds:**

   Target 1–2 small servings (a small palmful) per day. Almonds, sesame seeds (including tahini), chia, and pumpkin seeds give magnesium, plant protein, and unsaturated fats. Blend into oatmeal, add to salads, or use as a crunchy topping.

4. **Whole Grains:**

   Include whole grains at least twice daily: oats, quinoa, amaranth, buckwheat, whole grain bread, or brown rice bring magnesium, fiber, and B vitamins to support overall nutrient uptake and energy balance.

5. **Lean Protein Sources:**

   Plan for both animals (e.g., salmon, sardines, eggs, poultry) and plant sources (beans, lentils, tofu, tempeh) throughout the week. Fish with edible bones and eggs provide calcium plus vitamin D, while legumes and tofu bring magnesium and trace minerals.

6. **Colorful Vegetables and Fruits:**

   Fill one-third to half of each plate with a variety of vegetables and fruits (not just greens). Vitamin C, carotenoids, and bioactive compounds help reduce bone-resorbing inflammation and modulate mineral absorption.

When designing a meal, begin with your primary protein, add the major grain or starchy vegetable, layer on a green, and finish with nuts or seeds and a piece of fruit if desired.

## Portion Calibration Visual Plate Assembly Tool

Visual tools are helpful for keeping portions in check and ensuring nutrient-rich balance without weighing or measuring food every time. The following plate assembly method serves as a quick, repeatable guide for osteoporosis-supportive meals:

- ***Half Plate***: Non-starchy vegetables (with at least one serving leafy green per meal when possible). Examples: kale, spinach, peppers, carrots, broccoli.
- ***One Quarter Plate***: Protein source. Examples: grilled salmon, chicken breast, black beans, tofu, lentil patties.
- ***One Quarter Plate***: Whole grains or starchy root vegetables. Examples: quinoa, brown rice, millet, sweet potato, whole grain pasta.
- ***Side***: Calcium or vitamin D-fortified option. Include a cup of milk or its fortified alternative, or a small bowl of yogurt with ground seeds.
- ***Topping or Snack***: Handful of nuts/seeds, or a hard cheese slice.

Adjust this basic pattern for individual needs (energy expenditure, appetite, medical input), but use it as a consistent platform for meal-building. Over time, this visualization engrains optimal ratios and food group variety.

## Rotational Diversity Framework to Avoid Nutrient Monotony

Nutrient monotony relying on the same set of foods can sabotage micronutrient coverage, especially when trying to optimize bone health. Introducing a rotational diversity system creates natural dietary variety and maximizes the intake of lesser-known but vital nutrients.

**Key Elements of a Rotational Diversity Meal Framework:**

- ***Greens Rotation***: Switch main greens every other day (example: Monday - spinach; Tuesday - kale; Wednesday - bok choy, etc.).
- ***Protein Rotation***: Alternate between fish, poultry, vegetarian, and legume-based proteins over the week (e.g., salmon two days, lentils two days, chicken two days, tofu or tempeh on remaining day).
- ***Whole Grain Rotation***: Don't default to just one grain; cycle through oats, quinoa, brown rice, barley, amaranth, and buckwheat.
- ***Dairy/Fortified Alternative Rotation***: Include both cow's milk and different plant-fortified milks if tolerated, and use both soft and hard cheeses or their fortified vegan versions.

- ***Fruit and Vegetable Color Rotation***: Select across the spectrum—berries, citrus, apple, pear, melon, orange squash, red peppers, purple cabbage, green broccoli, yellow corn.
- ***Seed and Nut Rotation***: Change your seed (chia, pumpkin, sunflower) and nut (almond, walnut, pistachio, cashew) choice each day or week.

**Practicalities:**

- Post a weekly chart on the fridge listing "This Week's Rotations" for each food group.
- Use the outer aisles of the grocery store as your primary 'palette,' varying your picks seasonally as well.
- Plan main protein or grain components in your meal prep batch for several days, then swap to a new source to avoid repetition.

## Troubleshooting Guide for Vegetarian, Vegan, or Allergen-Avoidance Food Patterns

Even an optimized whole-food meal system can encounter hurdles from allergies, intolerances, ethical dietary choices, and medical conditions. Here, a troubleshooting matrix helps adapt your osteoporosis diet no matter the restriction.

**Dairy-Free or Vegan:**

- ***Dairy Substitutes***: Always choose calcium and vitamin D-fortified plant milks and yogurts (soy, almond, oat; check labels). Ensure protein intake with tofu, tempeh, lentils, and edamame; obtain vitamin K2 from fermented nondairy foods like natto if possible.
- ***Calcium Setbacks***: Fortified juices or firm tofu set with calcium sulfate may close the gap.
- ***Vitamin D Caution***: Consider mushrooms exposed to UV light, regularly include fortified foods, and discuss personalized supplements with your healthcare practitioner if food-based coverage is uncertain.

**Nut, Seed, or Soy Allergies:**

- ***Alternate Proteins***: Focus on beans, lentils, peas, eggs, fish, and poultry (if non-vegan); quinoa and amaranth for plant-based completeness.
- ***Fat Sources***: Use olive, avocado, or canola oil instead of nut/seed oils. Sunflower seed butters (for nut allergies) or dairy/egg may also work, depending on the allergy.
- ***Calcium***: Rely on leafy greens, canned (bone-in) fish if possible, and fortified grain products.

**Other Intolerances (Gluten, Nightshades):**

- ***Grains***: Use naturally gluten-free options (quinoa, buckwheat, rice, millet) if gluten is a concern.

- ***Vegetable Families***: Substitute non-nightshade veggies (such as greens, squash, carrots) if tomatoes, potatoes, or peppers aren't tolerated.

**Low Appetite or Digestive Issues:**

- Focus on smaller, more frequent meals; smooth blends (like smoothies or pureed soups) for ease of eating.
- Include calorie- and nutrient-dense snacks (yogurt, cheese, boiled eggs, seed butters) instead of low-calorie "empty" foods.

Every dietary pattern can be nutrient-complete for bone health with proactive adjustments and attention to fortified products where necessary.

A whole-food meal pattern that prioritizes variety, balance, and strategic planning is essential for lifelong bone health. By following these systems and adapting them to individual needs and preferences, you can ensure comprehensive nutrient coverage and prevent osteoporosis. With thoughtful meal design and regular adjustments, bone-supportive eating becomes a sustainable and rewarding habit.

# Shopping and Food Preparation Checklists for the Osteoporosis Diet (Tools)

For those managing or seeking to prevent osteoporosis, turning nutritional knowledge into real-world habits hinges on practical tools starting with how you shop, choose, store, and prepare food. While dietary principles define what's optimal for bone health, having concrete checklists and meal-building strategies ensures you consistently apply them. This chapter gives you step-by-step grocery guides, ingredient assessment tools, food storage insights, batch-cooking logistics, and practical meal formulas—helping you transform your kitchen into a foundation for lifelong bone strength.

## Step-by-Step Osteoporosis-Friendly Grocery List Template by Food Group

A smart grocery list is your first line of defense in building a bone-supportive pantry and refrigerator. By organizing your shopping by food group, you naturally streamline choices toward coverage of essential nutrients calcium, vitamin D, magnesium, protein, vitamin K2, and trace minerals.

**Divide your weekly list into these sections:**

1. **Dairy and Fortified Dairy Alternatives**
    - Milk, yogurt, kefir (cow's or calcium/vitamin D-fortified non-dairy alternatives—read labels for "fortified" not just "dairy-free")
    - Hard and soft cheeses (if tolerated)
    - Plant yogurts (look for both calcium and vitamin D fortification)
    - Calcium-set tofu

2. **Leafy Greens and Cruciferous Vegetables**
    - Spinach, kale, collards, bok choy, arugula
    - Broccoli, Brussels sprouts, cabbage

3. **Fish and Lean Protein Sources**
    - Salmon, sardines (especially canned with edible bones)
    - Eggs
    - Poultry (chicken, turkey)
    - Plant proteins: Lentils, chickpeas, black beans, edamame, tempeh

4. **Nuts, Seeds, and Related Products**
    - Almonds, walnuts, cashews, pistachios
    - Chia, pumpkin, sesame seeds

- Nut/seed butters (minimally processed; seek unsweetened varieties)

5. **Whole Grains and Starchy Roots**
    - Oats, quinoa, millet, amaranth, brown rice, buckwheat
    - Whole grain bread and pasta (look for 100% whole grain or "stone ground")
    - Sweet potatoes, carrots, parsnips

6. **Fruits and Colorful Vegetables**
    - Citrus (oranges, grapefruit), berries, apples, pears, cantaloupe
    - Red/orange/yellow peppers, squash, tomatoes, green beans

7. **Additional Nutrient Boosters**
    - Fortified orange juice (check nutrition label for calcium/vitamin D)
    - Dried mushrooms (UV-exposed for vitamin D, if available)
    - Herbs: parsley, basil, chives (Vitamin K-rich)
    - Avocados, olives (healthy fats)

8. **Miscellaneous Pantry Essentials**
    - Olive oil or avocado oil (for cooking, salad dressing)
    - Vinegar, lemon/lime juice (for flavor, without sodium)

- Low-sodium broth or stock
- Spices and salt-free seasoning blends

Keep a printed list or a template (digital or paper) in your kitchen, updating it weekly as you meal plan. Cross-reference your meal plan with your shopping list to avoid gaps that can lead to nutritional shortfalls.

## Ingredient Quality Checklist for Choosing Minimally Processed, Nutrient-Rich Items

Shopping for bone health isn't only about what you buy, but also the quality and processing level. Here's a quick checklist to help you select the highest-value food options for your osteoporosis diet:

- ☐ ***Prioritize whole and minimally processed foods***: opt for original forms (whole nuts, fresh vegetables, whole grains) over packages with long ingredient lists.
- ☐ ***Check the nutrition facts label*** for added sugars and sodium, especially in plant milks, yogurts, canned beans, and prepared grain products. Choose products with the lowest sodium and minimal or no added sugars.
- ☐ For dairy and plant milks/yogurts, ***read for "calcium-fortified" or "enriched with vitamin D."*** Look for products that provide at least 20–30% of daily value per serving.

- ☐ ***Avoid heavily fried, breaded, or ultra-processed protein sources***. Grilled, baked, poached, canned (in water), or plain are best.
- ☐ ***Select nuts and seeds*** that are raw or dry-roasted, unsalted, and not coated in excess oils or sugars.
- ☐ ***Choose whole grains*** in their complete form: "steel-cut" or "old-fashioned" oats, "whole grain" or "stone-ground" labels, and short ingredient lists.
- ☐ For fish, choose ***"wild-caught"*** if possible, and prioritize canned bone-in options for natural calcium.
- ☐ ***Avoid pre-seasoned*** or ready-to-eat vegetables and legumes that often contain excess salt.
- ☐ When buying juices or prepared foods, opt for those with ***"fortified with calcium/vitamin D"*** and without significant added sugars.

This checklist becomes second nature with practice. Use it as a filter before adding an item to your cart, whether in-store or shopping online.

## Seasonality and Storage Tables for Maximizing Nutrient Potency

Seasonality has a powerful influence on nutrient content, taste, and cost. In-season produce is often fresher, more affordable, and richer in vitamins and phytonutrients that support bone health. Equally important is how you store foods to maintain their nutritional quality until you eat them.

**Key Seasonal Choices for Osteoporosis Support:**

- ***Spring***: Asparagus, arugula, spinach, broccoli, peas, strawberries
- ***Summer***: Kale, collards, tomatoes, zucchini, berries, peaches, melons
- ***Fall***: Brussels sprouts, cabbage, turnips, squash, apples, pears, sweet potatoes
- ***Winter***: Cauliflower, carrots, leeks, parsnips, citrus fruits

**Storage Table (examples for nutrient freshness):**

- ***Leafy greens***: Store unwashed in a crisper, wrapped loosely in a paper towel and perforated bag; best within 3–5 days.
- ***Dairy/plant milk***: Refrigerate; use within a week after opening for best calcium/vitamin D content.
- ***Fish (canned)***: Store unopened in a cool pantry; refrigerate leftovers promptly and consume within 2 days.
- ***Nuts/seeds***: Store in airtight containers in the fridge or freezer to preserve healthy fats and vitamin E; use within 2–3 months.
- ***Whole grains***: Store uncooked grains in airtight containers in a cool, dry place; cooked grains keep in the refrigerator for up to 4 days or can be frozen for longer storage.

- ***Fruits and colorful vegetables***: Most do best in the fridge (except bananas, tomatoes, and potatoes); wash just before using.

## Batch Cooking and Advance Meal Prep Tools for Supporting Compliance

Batch cooking and preparing meals in advance are essential for maintaining dietary consistency, especially when time or energy is limited. Organizations and tools that streamline prep mean you're far more likely to meet your bone nutrient needs each day.

**Essential Tools for Advance Prep:**

- Large-capacity pots and sauté pans for making stews, soups, and grains in bulk
- Sheet pans for roasting multiple trays of vegetables and proteins at once
- Food processor or high-speed blender for chopping, pureeing, or blending smoothies and spreads
- Storage containers in assorted sizes (preferably glass or BPA-free plastic) for leftovers, pre-portioned snacks, and ready-to-go lunches
- Measuring cups/spoons and food scale (for initial learning, though visual cues become sufficient with practice)
- Rice cooker or multicooker automates whole grain, bean, or soup batch prep

**Batch Cooking Strategies:**

- Double or triple staple recipes (chili, lentil stew, quinoa pilaf, baked chicken or tofu) and freeze in individual meal portions.
- Wash and chop snack veggies (carrots, celery, bell peppers) and leafy greens at the start of the week, storing them in visible, easy-to-grab containers.
- Prepare overnight oats or soaked chia puddings for no-cook, calcium-protein-rich breakfasts.
- Pre-cook whole grains and beans; use throughout the week in grain bowls, soups, salads, and stir-fries.
- Hard-boil eggs for grab-and-go snacks or meal add-ons.
- Portion nuts/seeds into single-serve bags or containers to avoid over-eating but ensure coverage.

Consistency in prepping bone-building foods guarantees that each day, regardless of schedule, classically important foods are consumed.

## Simple Meal-Building Formula for Quick, Balanced Osteoporosis-Appropriate Dishes

Once your pantry and refrigerator are stocked, meal-building should be fast and intuitive. Use this "1-2-3-4" formula to ensure every meal has the power to protect your bones:

1. **Choose One Protein Source**

   Eggs, beans, lentils, fish, tofu, chicken, or Greek yogurt

2. **Add Two Vibrant Vegetables**

   Include a leafy green and a second color for anti-inflammatory and micronutrient variety (e.g., spinach + red bell pepper; kale + orange squash)

3. **Select a Grain or Starchy Vegetable**

   Quinoa, oats, brown rice, millet, whole grain bread, or sweet potato

4. **Include a Bone-Boosting Bonus**

   Dairy or fortified plant milk, a small square of calcium-fortified tofu, or a handful of nuts or seeds

**Example Quick Meals:**

- ***Breakfast***: Greek yogurt (protein) + berries (color) + spinach (green) + sprinkle of walnuts (bonus)
- ***Lunch***: Lentil soup (protein) with kale (green) and carrots (color), side of whole grain bread, small glass of fortified soy milk
- ***Dinner***: Baked salmon (protein), roasted broccoli (green) and red pepper (color), quinoa, slice of cheese (bonus)

- ***Snacks***: Cottage cheese and pineapple, hummus with raw veggies, fortified almond milk smoothie with frozen berries and pea protein.

Using this pattern, you can build hundreds of osteoporosis-supportive meals with zero guesswork.

With these tools, checklists, and answers, you're equipped to confidently shop, store, cook, and assemble meals that move beyond theoretical nutrition directly serving your bone health, every day.

# 7-Day Sample Meal Plans with Nutrient Highlights (Examples)

Designing weekly meal plans that nurture bone health is the bridge between osteoporosis diet principles and sustained dietary behavior. This chapter provides a full seven-day sample meal plan, each day parsed by key nutrients calcium, vitamin D, magnesium, protein, and other bone-protective elements.

To help you personalize further, you'll find a substitution matrix to swap main items according to taste or dietary requirements, a timing guide for meal and snack spacing that maximizes nutrient absorption, a color-coded chart that serves as a visual prompt for dietary diversity, and a clear tracking sheet for adherence and self-assessment.

## Complete 7-Day Sample Meal Plan with Nutrient Highlights

Below you'll find a comprehensive osteoporosis-supportive meal plan. Each entry highlights protein, calcium, vitamin D, magnesium, and color variety, helping ensure all critical nutrients for bone health are covered. The foods selected are minimally processed, incorporate fortified alternatives as needed, and build on the "1-2-3-4" meal formula already described.

**Day 1**

***Breakfast***: Greek yogurt parfait with mixed berries, spinach, and chia seeds

***Snack***: Cottage cheese with pineapple

***Lunch***: Lentil and kale soup, whole grain toast, orange slices

***Snack***: Raw almonds, carrot sticks

***Dinner***: Baked salmon, roasted broccoli and sweet potato, small glass of calcium-fortified soy milk

**Daily Highlights:**

- ***Protein***: Greek yogurt, lentils, salmon, soy milk
- ***Calcium***: Yogurt, cottage cheese, fortified milk, almonds
- ***Vitamin D***: Salmon, fortified soy milk
- ***Magnesium***: Chia seeds, almonds, whole grains, leafy greens
- ***Color variety***: Berries (red/blue), spinach (green), carrots (orange), sweet potato (orange), broccoli (green), orange fruit

**Day 2**

***Breakfast***: Oatmeal with fortified almond milk, walnuts, blueberries

***Snack***: Hard-boiled egg

***Lunch***: Chickpea and spinach salad with red peppers, feta, whole wheat pita

***Snack***: Pumpkin seeds, apple

***Dinner***: Sardines on whole grain crackers, steamed green beans, quinoa pilaf

**Highlights:**

- ***Protein***: Egg, chickpeas, sardines
- ***Calcium***: Fortified milk, feta, sardines (with bones)
- ***Vitamin D***: Sardines, fortified almond milk
- ***Magnesium***: Walnuts, pumpkin seeds, quinoa
- ***Color***: Blueberries, red pepper, green beans, apple

**Day 3**

***Breakfast***: Scrambled eggs with kale and tomatoes, whole grain English muffin

***Snack***: Calcium-set tofu cubes with cucumber

***Lunch***: Turkey and roasted vegetable wrap, side of kiwi

***Snack***: Sesame sticks, baby bell peppers

***Dinner***: Grilled trout, sautéed Swiss chard, brown rice, glass of fortified orange juice

**Highlights:**

- ***Protein***: Eggs, tofu, turkey, trout
- ***Calcium***: Tofu, Swiss chard, fortified OJ
- ***Vitamin D***: Trout, fortified OJ
- ***Magnesium***: Kale, whole grains, sesame sticks
- ***Color***: Tomatoes (red), chard (green), kiwi (green), bell peppers (red/yellow)

**Day 4**

***Breakfast***: Fortified soy yogurt with granola and fresh strawberries

***Snack***: String cheese, clementine

***Lunch***: Tuna salad over arugula with avocado and pumpkin seeds, whole grain roll

***Snack***: Edamame, pear

***Dinner***: Baked chicken breast, Brussels sprouts, roasted parsnip and carrots

**Highlights:**

- ***Protein***: Soy yogurt, tuna, chicken, edamame
- ***Calcium***: Soy yogurt, string cheese, arugula, Brussels sprouts

- ***Vitamin D***: Tuna, fortified soy yogurt
- ***Magnesium***: Pumpkin seeds, avocado, whole grains
- ***Color***: Strawberries, clementine (orange), parsnip/ carrots (yellow/orange), avocado (green)

**Day 5**

***Breakfast***: Overnight oats with chia, fortified soy milk, and sliced banana

***Snack***: Boiled egg, cherry tomatoes

***Lunch***: Black bean chili with bell peppers, corn, and cilantro, side of brown rice

***Snack***: Hummus and red pepper strips

***Dinner***: Broiled mackerel, sautéed collard greens, baked potato, glass of kefir

**Highlights:**

- ***Protein***: Soy milk, egg, beans, mackerel
- ***Calcium***: Soy milk, collards, kefir
- ***Vitamin D***: Mackerel, kefir, fortified soy milk
- ***Magnesium***: Chia, black beans, greens
- ***Color***: Banana (yellow), tomatoes (red), peppers (mixed), collard greens (green), potato (brown/white)

**Day 6**

***Breakfast***: Whole grain toast with almond butter, sliced pear

***Snack***: Low-fat kefir smoothie with spinach, mango, and pea protein

***Lunch***: Quinoa and roasted vegetable bowl with chickpeas, tahini dressing

***Snack***: Cottage cheese, kiwi

***Dinner***: Tofu stir-fry with bok choy, mushrooms, and bell peppers, served over brown rice

**Highlights:**

- ***Protein***: Almond butter, pea protein, cottage cheese, tofu, chickpeas
- ***Calcium***: Kefir, tahini, bok choy, cottage cheese
- ***Vitamin D***: Fortified kefir, UV-exposed mushrooms
- ***Magnesium***: Almond butter, spinach, whole grains
- ***Color***: Mango (yellow), spinach (green), bell peppers (mixed), bok choy (green)

**Day 7**

***Breakfast***: Smoothie bowl (fortified soy milk, berries, flaxseed, kale) topped with granola

***Snack***: Roasted chickpeas, orange slices

***Lunch***: Grilled shrimp salad with mixed greens, avocado, pumpkin seeds

***Snack***: Greek yogurt, blueberries

***Dinner***: Baked tilapia, roasted sweet potato, steamed broccoli

**Highlights:**

- ***Protein***: Soy milk, chickpeas, shrimp, Greek yogurt, tilapia
- ***Calcium***: Soy milk, yogurt, pumpkin seeds, broccoli
- ***Vitamin D***: Fortified soy milk, tilapia
- ***Magnesium***: Flaxseed, pumpkin seeds, greens
- ***Color***: Berries (red/blue), kale (green), mixed greens, sweet potato (orange), blueberries

**Daily Nutrient Totals (Approximated, may vary with portion size and specific brand/fortification):**

- ***Protein***: 75-90g
- ***Calcium***: 1000-1300mg
- ***Vitamin D***: 400-700 IU (higher with adequate use of fortified foods or oily fish)
- ***Magnesium***: 350-450mg
- ***Notable variety***: At least 4 distinct color groups per day for phytonutrient diversity

## Substitution Guide for Individualizing Meal Plans

To maximize compliance and enjoyment, tailor meals to your requirements using the following:

1. **Protein Alternatives:**
   - Swap Greek yogurt ↔ fortified soy yogurt
   - Replace any fish dish with baked tofu or calcium-set tempeh (for vegetarians)
   - Substitute poultry with legumes or lentil-based products

2. **Dairy/Fortified Dairy Alternatives:**
   - Use fortified almond or oat milk in place of cow's or soy milk if allergy/sensitivity
   - For cheese: try low-sodium, plant-based cheese made with added calcium

3. **Vegetable Diversity:**
   - Substitute any leafy green (kale, spinach, collard, chard) with bok choy, arugula, or romaine
   - Mix cruciferous (broccoli, Brussels sprouts) with cauliflower or cabbage

4. **Grain and Starchy Sides:**
   - Swap quinoa ↔ millet, farro, or amaranth
   - Swap brown rice ↔ bulgur or barley
   - Gluten-free: Use certified GF oats, brown rice, sweet potato instead of wheat-based products

5. **Snack Customization:**
   - Nuts/seeds: Swap almonds with walnuts, pumpkin seeds with sunflower seeds

- For high-protein/low dairy: Use roasted chickpeas, edamame, or protein-rich smoothies

6. **Fruit Choices:**

   Choose in-season fruits for higher vitamin content and cost savings

**Other:**

- ***For vegan diets***: Exclude eggs and fish, using more legumes and fortified plant foods
- ***For allergies***: Eliminate the offending ingredient and substitute with an equivalent nutrient value

## Timeline for Meal and Snack Spacing to Optimize Uptake

Properly spaced meals and snacks can help the body maximize use of bone-building nutrients like calcium, magnesium, and protein:

- ***Breakfast***: Within 1 hour of waking for protein and calcium replenishment
- ***Mid-Morning Snack***: 2-3 hours after breakfast to maintain energy and calcium status
- ***Lunch***: Midday, positioned 3-4 hours after breakfast—combines protein and a fresh array of vegetables/whole grains
- ***Afternoon Snack***: 2-3 hours after lunch, supporting sustained muscle and bone repair before dinner

- ***Dinner***: 3-4 hours after lunch; should not be rushed to maximize protein digestion and absorption of minerals
- ***Optional***: Light, protein-rich snack before bed if overall daily protein or calcium intake remains low

**Tips for maximizing nutrient absorption and minimizing antagonism:**

- Avoid pairing high-oxalate foods (like spinach) exclusively as your only calcium source; rotate other greens to diversify intake
- Separate calcium-rich foods from high-iron supplements by at least two hours to prevent mineral competition
- Spread total protein and calcium across the day rather than concentrating at one meal
- Vitamin D-rich foods (fish/fatty meals, fortified products) are best absorbed with some dietary fat, so include oils or nuts

### Visual Reference Chart: Meal Color Spectrum and Nutrient Coverage

A colorful plate often reflects a nutrient-dense meal. Use this quick guide to spot missing color groups and improve micro- and phytonutrient variety.

Table 6: Visual Reference Chart

| Color Group | Key Food Examples | Notable Nutrients |
|---|---|---|
| Green | Kale, spinach, broccoli, bok choy | Vitamin K, magnesium, potassium, folate |
| Orange/Yellow | Sweet potato, carrots, bell peppers, mango | Beta-carotene (vitamin A), vitamin C, antioxidants |
| Red/Purple | Berries, tomatoes, grapes, red cabbage | Vitamin C, anthocyanins, polyphenols, lycopene |
| White/Brown | Tofu, beans, oats, dairy, mushrooms | Protein, calcium, vitamin D (if fortified), fiber, selenium |

**Tip**: Aim for at least three different color groups at each main meal and four or more across the day to help ensure broad nutrient coverage.

Example:

- ***Breakfast***: Green (spinach), red (berries), white (yogurt)
- ***Lunch***: Green (kale), orange (carrot), brown (whole grain bread)
- ***Dinner***: White (fish), green (broccoli), orange (sweet potato)

## Compliance Tracking Sheet: Weekly Assessment and Adjustment

To ensure adherence and identify improvement areas, use a simple compliance tracker. Review and check each box as you fulfill each day's nutrient goals and recommended variety:

**Daily Tracker (Example)**

- ☐ 3+ servings of high-quality protein
- ☐ 3+ servings of calcium-rich foods (dairy or fortified alternatives, tofu, leafy greens)
- ☐ 1+ vitamin D–rich food (oily fish, fortified product, or UV-exposed mushrooms)
- ☐ 2+ servings whole grains or starchy root vegetables
- ☐ 1+ serving nuts or seeds
- ☐ 4+ color groups represented in meals
- ☐ No more than 1 high-sodium or ultra-processed item
- ☐ Snacks are nutrient-dense and minimally processed
- ☐ Meals and snacks spaced every 2–4 hours

**Weekly Review:**

- Mark days when all boxes are checked
- Tally and review triggers for missed categories (e.g., running out of healthy snacks, skipping fortified foods, not rotating vegetables)
- Adjust next week's plan for weak spots for example, pre-chopping more greens, prepping extra fish or plant protein, or trying new fortified products

Implementing a thoughtfully structured meal plan can make a significant difference in supporting bone health and preventing osteoporosis. With diverse, nutrient-rich foods and flexible substitutions, these guidelines are designed to fit a variety of tastes and dietary needs. Regularly tracking your choices empowers you to make informed adjustments and build lasting, bone-strengthening habits.

# Bone-Building Recipes with Stepwise Preparations

Unlocking the potential of an osteoporosis-specific diet means moving from theory to action preparing meals that are flavorful, appealing, and optimized for bone health. This chapter provides you with expertly curated recipes, each specifically designed to deliver the essential nutrients your bones need.

Every recipe is tagged for its key nutrient focus (e.g., calcium-rich, vitamin D-enhanced, magnesium-packed, or plant-based protein), and matched to a culinary skill level from beginner to intermediate. To foster long-term adherence, you'll also find practical substitution options for allergies, intolerances, or dietary preferences, along with tips for efficient workflow and attractive presentation. Comprehensive nutrient breakdowns accompany each dish, empowering you to align meal choices with your daily bone-building targets.

## Recipe Cards for High-Nutrient Dishes

The following recipes are organized by nutrient emphasis and culinary skill level, facilitating selection based on your nutritional goals and kitchen confidence. Each is crafted to align with osteoporosis nutrition principles and can serve as a template for ongoing meal planning.

## Greek Yogurt Breakfast Parfait

**Focus**: High Calcium & Protein

**Skill Level**: Beginner

**Ingredients:**

- Greek yogurt
- Mixed berries
- Chia seeds
- Chopped almonds

**Instructions:**

1. In a cup or bowl, add a layer of Greek yogurt.
2. Add a layer of mixed berries on top of the yogurt.
3. Sprinkle chia seeds and chopped almonds over the berries.
4. Repeat layers if desired.
5. Chill for 5 minutes before serving. Enjoy!

**Nutrient Snapshot:**

***Calcium***: 250mg/serving

***Protein***: 15g/serving

***Magnesium***: 40mg/serving.

## Savory Lentil & Kale Soup

**Focus**: Magnesium & Plant Protein

**Skill Level**: Beginner

**Ingredients:**

- Dry green lentils
- Chopped kale
- Carrots
- Celery
- Onion
- Garlic
- Low-sodium broth

**Instructions:**

1. In a large pot, sauté chopped onion and minced garlic until fragrant.
2. Add chopped carrots and celery, and cook for a few minutes until slightly softened.
3. Pour in the low-sodium broth and add dry green lentils.
4. Bring to a boil, then lower heat and simmer for about 30 minutes, or until lentils are tender.
5. Stir in chopped kale during the last few minutes of cooking.
6. Adjust seasoning as needed and serve hot.

**Nutrient Snapshot:**

***Protein***: 10g/serving

***Magnesium***: 50mg/serving,

***Potassium***: 400mg/serving.

## Calcium-Set Tofu Stir-Fry with Bok Choy

**Focus**: Calcium, Magnesium, Plant Protein

**Skill Level**: Intermediate

**Ingredients:**

- Firm calcium-set tofu
- Bok choy
- Bell peppers
- Soy sauce
- Sesame oil

**Instructions:**

1. Cut the tofu into cubes and pat dry with a paper towel.
2. Heat sesame oil in a large skillet or wok over medium-high heat.
3. Add the tofu cubes and stir-fry until golden on all sides.
4. Add chopped bok choy and sliced bell peppers to the pan.
5. Stir-fry until the vegetables are tender.
6. Add soy sauce to taste, toss to combine, and serve hot.

**Nutrient Snapshot:**

***Calcium***: 250mg/serving

***Protein***: 12g,

***Vitamin*** K: (high),

***Magnesium***: 40mg.

## Grilled Salmon with Roasted Broccoli

**Focus**: Vitamin D & Omega-3s

**Skill Level**: Beginner

**Ingredients:**

- Salmon fillets
- Broccoli florets
- Olive oil
- Lemon

**Instructions:**

1. Preheat the oven to 400°F (200°C).
2. Place salmon fillets and broccoli florets on a baking sheet.
3. Brush both salmon and broccoli with olive oil.
4. Roast in the oven for 20 minutes until salmon is cooked through and broccoli is tender.
5. Squeeze fresh lemon juice over the salmon and broccoli just before serving.

**Nutrient Snapshot:**

***Vitamin D***: 20mcg (if wild)

***Protein***: 23g

***Magnesium***: 25mg

## Oatmeal with Fortified Almond Milk and Walnuts

**Focus**: Calcium, Magnesium, Plant Protein

**Skill Level**: Beginner

**Ingredients:**

- Rolled oats
- Fortified almond milk
- Chopped walnuts
- Blueberries

**Instructions:**

1. In a saucepan, cook rolled oats in fortified almond milk according to package directions.
2. Once cooked, transfer the oatmeal to a bowl.
3. Top with chopped walnuts and blueberries.
4. Serve warm and enjoy.

**Nutrient Snapshot:**

***Calcium***: 250mg,

***Magnesium***: 60mg

## Sardines on Whole Grain Crackers

**Focus**: Calcium & Vitamin D

**Skill Level**: Beginner

**Ingredients:**

- Tinned sardines in water/oil (with bones)
- Whole-grain crackers
- Arugula

**Instructions:**

1. Arrange whole-grain crackers on a plate.
2. Place sardines (with bones) on top of each cracker.
3. Top each sardine with a few leaves of arugula.

**Nutrient Snapshot:**

***Calcium***: 300mg/serving,

***Vitamin D***: 4-6mcg/serving.

## Scrambled Eggs with Spinach and Tomatoes

***Focus***: Protein, Vitamin K

***Skill Level***: Beginner

**Ingredients:**

- Eggs
- Spinach
- Cherry tomatoes
- Black pepper

**Instructions:**

1. Heat a nonstick pan over medium heat.
2. Add spinach and cook until wilted.
3. Beat the eggs in a bowl and pour them into the pan.
4. Add cherry tomatoes, sliced in half.
5. Gently scramble the mixture until eggs are cooked through.
6. Season with black pepper to taste.

**Nutrient Snapshot:**

***Protein***: 4g/2 eggs,

***Vitamin K***: (high)

## Vegetable and Chickpea Curry

**Focus**: Plant Protein, Magnesium

**Skill Level**: Intermediate

**Ingredients:**

- Chickpeas
- Onion
- Bell pepper
- Diced tomato
- Spinach
- Curry powder

**Instructions:**

1. Heat a large pan over medium heat and sauté chopped onion and bell pepper until softened.
2. Add diced tomatoes, chickpeas, spinach, and curry powder to the pan.
3. Stir well to combine all ingredients.
4. Simmer the mixture for 20 minutes, stirring occasionally.

**Nutrient Snapshot:**

***Protein***: 10g/serving,

***Magnesium***: 45mg.

## Black Bean Chili

**Focus**: Plant Protein, Fiber, Magnesium

**Skill Level**: Intermediate

**Ingredients:**

- Black beans
- Diced tomatoes
- Corn
- Bell pepper
- Cumin
- Onion

**Instructions:**

1. In a large pot, sauté diced onion and bell pepper until soft.
2. Add black beans, diced tomatoes, corn, and cumin.
3. Stir to combine, then bring to a simmer.
4. Simmer for 30 minutes, stirring occasionally.

**Nutrient Snapshot:**

***Protein***: 12g

***Magnesium***: 60mg

***Fiber***: ~6g.

## Baked Mackerel with Sweet Potato

**Focus**: Vitamin D & Omega-3

**Skill Level**: Intermediate

**Ingredients:**

- Mackerel fillet
- Sweet potato
- Olive oil

**Instructions:**

1. Preheat the oven to 400°F (200°C).
2. Slice the sweet potato into rounds or wedges and place on a baking sheet.
3. Drizzle sweet potato slices with olive oil.
4. Place the mackerel fillet on the baking sheet alongside the sweet potato.
5. Bake for 20 minutes, or until the mackerel is cooked through and the sweet potato is tender.

**Nutrient Snapshot:**

***Vitamin D***: 15mcg/fillet,

***Magnesium***: 35mg.

## Low-Fat Kefir Smoothie with Spinach and Mango

**Focus**: Calcium, Vitamin D, Probiotics

**Skill Level**: Beginner

**Ingredients:**

- Low-fat kefir
- Spinach
- Mango chunks
- Ice

**Instructions:**

1. Add low-fat kefir, spinach, mango chunks, and ice to a blender.
2. Blend on high until the mixture is completely smooth.

**Nutrient Snapshot:**

***Calcium***: 250mg,

***Vitamin D***: 3mcg

***Vitamin C***: (high)

## Quinoa & Roasted Vegetable Bowl

**Focus**: Magnesium, Plant Protein

**Skill Level**: Intermediate

**Ingredients:**

- Quinoa
- Zucchini
- Carrots
- Bell peppers
- Olive oil

**Instructions:**

1. Preheat the oven and chop zucchini, carrots, and bell peppers.
2. Toss vegetables with olive oil and roast until tender.
3. Cook quinoa according to package instructions.
4. Combine roasted vegetables and quinoa, drizzle with a bit more olive oil if desired.

**Nutrient Snapshot:**

***Magnesium***: 50mg,

***Protein***: 8g.

## Greek Yogurt Dip with Crudités

**Focus**: Calcium, Protein, Vitamin C

**Skill Level**: Beginner

**Ingredients:**

- Greek yogurt
- Lemon juice
- Chopped dill
- Assorted vegetables (for dipping)

**Instructions:**

1. In a bowl, mix Greek yogurt, lemon juice, and chopped dill until well combined.
2. Serve the dip with a platter of cut vegetables.

**Nutrient Snapshot:**

***Calcium***: 150mg,

***Vitamin C***: (by vegetables).

## Tofu and Edamame Salad

**Focus**: Plant Protein, Iron, Calcium

**Skill Level**: Beginner

**Ingredients:**

- Cubed tofu
- Shelled edamame
- Shredded carrot
- Sesame seeds
- Low-sodium soy sauce

**Instructions:**

1. In a large bowl, combine cubed tofu, shelled edamame, and shredded carrot.
2. Sprinkle with sesame seeds and drizzle with low-sodium soy sauce.
3. Toss well to combine and serve cold.

**Nutrient Snapshot:**

***Protein***: 18g/serving

***Calcium***: 200mg

***Magnesium***: 40mg.

## Fortified Soy Yogurt with Berry Compote

**Focus**: Calcium, Vitamin D, Antioxidants

**Skill Level**: Beginner

**Ingredients:**

- Fortified soy yogurt
- Mixed berries
- Honey

**Instructions:**

1. In a small saucepan, simmer mixed berries with a drop of honey until a compote forms.
2. Spoon the berry compote over the fortified soy yogurt.

**Nutrient Snapshot:**

***Calcium***: 200mg

***Vitamin D***: 2mcg

***Polyphenols***: (berries).

## Ingredient Substitution Guide

Creating osteoporosis-friendly recipes shouldn't mean restricting variety due to allergies or personal preferences. Use the following substitution options to tailor dishes while preserving nutrient profiles:

**Dairy-free / Lactose Intolerance:**

- Swap cow's milk yogurt for fortified soy or almond yogurt.
- Use lactose-free milk or fortified plant milks for all oatmeal, smoothie, or cereal-based recipes.
- Hard cheeses (e.g., cheddar) are often tolerated and lower in lactose.
- Explore calcium-set tofu and fortified non-dairy cheeses as additional sources.

**Vegan/Vegetarian:**

- Replace fish and poultry with firm tofu, tempeh, lentils, or beans in mains.
- Omit eggs; increase beans, nuts, or add vegan protein powders.
- Select fortified plant milks, yogurts, and spreads for calcium and vitamin D needs.

**Nut Allergies:**

- Substitute seeds (sunflower, pumpkin) for nuts in all toppings or mixes.

- Use tahini for creamy dressings in place of nut butter.

**Gluten-Free:**

Use certified gluten-free oats, brown rice, quinoa, or sweet potato in place of wheat-based grains in any recipe.

**Allergy to Soy:**

Use dairy or pea protein yogurts, replace tofu/edamame with lentils, chickpeas, or eggs.

## Stepwise Kitchen Workflow For Efficiency

Maximizing time in the kitchen doesn't require expert skills, just strategic steps:

1. Gather all ingredients, measuring and prepping (washing, chopping, soaking) before you turn on the stove.
2. Start with foods that require the longest cook time (e.g., roasting or boiling vegetables, baking fish or poultry).
3. While the main components cook, assemble salads, prepare dips, and set cold garnishes.
4. Batch-cook grains (quinoa, rice, oats) early in the week for quick use in multiple recipes .
5. Clean as you go to keep the workspace clear and speed up post-cooking tasks.

6. When making smoothies or salads, chop extra greens and vegetables for storage—these keep well and simplify assembling nutritious meals later.

### Plate Presentation Tips for Enhanced Appeal

Appealing meals help reinforce adherence to dietary routines. Try these techniques:

- Use a palette of at least three colors per plate, think green leafy vegetables, orange sweet potato, and red peppers for visual appeal and nutrient diversity.
- Stack elements in contrasting layers (e.g., yogurt beneath berries and nuts; roasted fish atop bright greens).
- Garnish simply with fresh herbs (dill, parsley) or a twist of lemon for freshness.
- Arrange bowls with a mix of textures (creamy, crunchy, soft) to make plant-rich dishes visually enticing.
- Serve dips in small ramekins, vegetables in wedges or strips, and proteins sliced neatly for professional flair.

## Nutrient Breakdown Charts by Recipe

The table below offers a quick reference for major nutrient deliveries by recipe (per standard serving):

Table 7: Nutrient Breakdown Charts

| Recipe Name | Calcium (mg) | Vit D (mcg) | Protein (g) | Magnesium (mg) | Vit K | Fiber (g) |
|---|---|---|---|---|---|---|
| Greek Yogurt Parfait | ~250 | 0 | 15 | 40 | ✓ | 3 |
| Lentil & Kale Soup | 40 | 0 | 10 | 50 | ✓ | 5 |
| Tofu Stir-Fry with Bok Choy | ~250 | 0 | 12 | 40 | ✓ | 4 |
| Grilled Salmon & Roasted Broccoli | 35 | 20 | 23 | 25 | ✓ | 3 |
| Oatmeal with Fortified Almond Milk | ~250 | 2 | 6 | 60 | | 4 |
| Sardines on Whole Grain Crackers | 300 | 6 | 12 | 40 | | 2 |
| Scrambled Eggs with Spinach | 70 | 2 | 14 | 20 | ✓ | 2 |
| Vegetable & Chickpea Curry | 90 | 0 | 10 | 45 | | 6 |
| Black Bean Chili | 75 | 0 | 12 | 60 | | 6 |
| Baked Mackerel with Sweet Potato | 30 | 15 | 20 | 35 | | 3 |
| Kefir Smoothie with Spinach/ Mango | 250 | 3 | 10 | 30 | ✓ | 2 |
| Quinoa & Roasted Veg Bowl | 40 | 0 | 8 | 50 | ✓ | 5 |
| Yogurt Dip with Crudités | 150 | 0 | 6 | 15 | | 3+ |
| Tofu & Edamame Salad | 200 | 0 | | | | |

These recipes offer a practical and enjoyable way to support bone health through everyday meals. With nutrient-focused tags and adaptable options for various dietary needs, you can easily tailor dishes to your preferences. The workflow and presentation tips help make meal preparation efficient and visually appealing. Use the nutrient breakdowns to confidently plan and track your bone-building nutrition.

# Conclusion

The Osteoporosis Diet Guide has walked you through a comprehensive, stepwise approach to supporting bone health with nutrition demonstrating that effective dietary management extends far beyond simply meeting calcium requirements. As you put this knowledge into action, it's valuable to integrate the four-step bone-building framework seamlessly with practical shopping, planning, and preparation habits to foster lasting change.

To begin, anchor your bone-healthy lifestyle with a sequenced action plan. Start each week by revisiting the meal planning tools, selecting recipes and grocery staples from your provided checklists, and building a shopping list that focuses on whole, minimally processed foods rich in protein, vitamin D, vitamin K2, magnesium, and supportive trace minerals.

Allocate a window for batch preparation of core ingredients such as cooked grains, pre-washed greens, and ready-to-eat proteins so that assembling balanced meals becomes routine instead of overwhelming. For daily execution, employ simple visual cues: plate assembly templates and food group prioritization rules ensure that each meal covers all critical nutrient bases. This approach not only provides structure but also relieves decision fatigue, making it far more likely that you will stick with the plan over time.

By adhering consistently to these strategies, you can expect measurable improvements in dietary quality, which is proven to favorably shape your long-term bone health trajectory. The 4-step system—centered on optimizing protein intake, ensuring sufficient vitamins and minerals, limiting bone-depleting foods, and constructing whole-food patterns acts synergistically to address multiple modifiable risk factors for osteoporosis simultaneously. However, it's important to recognize the boundaries of this approach.

Dietary changes operate within individual physiological variations and should always complement, not replace, routine medical oversight and bone density monitoring. Certain medications, health conditions, or advanced stages of osteoporosis may warrant additional interventions, so maintain open communication with your healthcare provider regarding your nutrition plan.

For ongoing success, embrace a mindset of steady adjustment and monitoring. Use the meal and compliance trackers provided in this guide to regularly review both your nutrient intake and the diversity of foods selected throughout the weeks. Rotating recipes, seasonal ingredients, and food group sources can help prevent both menu fatigue and micronutrient shortfalls. Should you notice lapses in preparing balanced meals, return to the troubleshooting checklists: review storage solutions, refresh your kitchen mise en place, or schedule time for freezer-friendly batch cooking to reclaim convenience. To stay motivated, celebrate small wins—such as successfully introducing a new high-magnesium recipe or consistently limiting high-sodium foods—and consider setting periodic reminders for dietary reassessment or adaptive changes as your needs evolve.

In summary, sustaining bone health through nutrition is an ongoing process unified by preparation, planning, and mindful meal execution. Whether you are newly diagnosed with osteoporosis or aiming for prevention, the steps and tools in this guide equip you to act proactively—nourishing your body with intention and supporting your bones at every stage of life. By following this system over the long term, you cultivate a dietary routine that is feasible, enjoyable, and fundamentally restorative for your skeletal health.

# FAQs

## How should I adjust my meal plan based on my osteoporosis diagnosis?

Osteoporosis is not a one-size-fits-all diagnosis, and diet should evolve with your stage and bone density. If you have low bone mass (osteopenia), prioritize nutrients like calcium, vitamin D, magnesium, and protein, while reducing foods high in salt, sugar, and caffeine. Focus on more calcium- and vitamin D-rich foods, such as low-fat dairy, leafy greens, and fortified plant-based alternatives. Regular protein intake at every meal supports bone turnover.

With an osteoporosis diagnosis or history of fractures, further customization is needed. Adjust portion sizes, spread out nutrient-rich foods to align with medication schedules, and consider easily digestible, high-nutrient meals. You may benefit from more frequent snacks and should avoid exceeding safe upper limits for nutrients. Consult your healthcare provider to refine nutrient targets as your bone status changes.

**Can I follow the osteoporosis diet if I am dairy-free, lactose intolerant, vegetarian, or plant-based?**

Absolutely. The main goal is to maximize bone-protective nutrients, which can be found in non-dairy and plant-based sources. Prioritize calcium-rich foods like collard greens, bok choy, almonds, sesame seeds, figs, and calcium-fortified plant milks or tofu. For vitamin D, rely on sunlight, fortified foods, and UV-exposed mushrooms. Plant-based diets should include a variety of beans, lentils, soy products, nuts, seeds, and whole grains for protein. Regular reviews with a health professional can help monitor for nutritional gaps.

**How can I safely incorporate supplements with my osteoporosis diet?**

Supplements, especially calcium and vitamin D, can be important but must be used carefully. First, assess your dietary intake with a food diary or tracker. Discuss supplement use and possible blood tests with your healthcare provider. Do not exceed recommended daily allowances unless advised. For calcium, total intake should not exceed 1200 mg per day for most adults; vitamin D's upper limit is typically 4000 IU daily.

Take calcium supplements in divided doses for best absorption, and be mindful of interactions with medications. Watch for side effects like digestive discomfort or signs of excess, and consult your medical team as needed.

### Which foods should I include or avoid to counteract medication side effects affecting bones?

Some osteoporosis or other medications can harm bone health. Include calcium-rich foods (leafy greens, low-fat dairy or fortified alternatives, tofu, almonds, canned fish with bones), vitamin D-fortified foods, magnesium- and potassium-rich plant foods (nuts, seeds, legumes, avocados, bananas), and high-protein foods (lean meats, eggs, legumes, soy). Limit sodium (processed foods, canned soups), sugary items, excess caffeine (under 400 mg daily), and alcohol. Your doctor or dietitian can advise if medication changes nutrient needs.

### How do I maintain my osteoporosis diet when dining out or traveling?

Plan ahead: check menus for calcium, protein, and veggie-rich options. Choose nutrient-dense meals, request reduced-sodium preparations, and bring portable snacks like nuts, calcium-fortified bars, or instant oatmeal. Choose water or unsweetened plant milks over sugary drinks, and don't skip meals. Communicate dietary needs to restaurants and, when traveling, stock up on essentials at grocery stores.

### What common diet pitfalls could jeopardize bone strength?

Watch for very low-calorie diets, which can cause nutrient shortages and bone loss. Even plant-based diets can miss calcium or protein if not carefully planned. Avoid excess sodium in processed foods, too much caffeine, and strict fat avoidance healthy fats help absorb vitamins vital for bones. Avoid unproven diet trends that neglect core bone nutrients.

**How should I track my bone health as I change my diet?**

Regular bone density testing (DEXA/DXA scans), blood tests for vitamin D and calcium, and keeping a food diary are important. Note any new bone pain or falls, and review medications and supplements with your provider at least annually or when situations change. This helps you adjust your diet and supplement plan to support your bone health.

The osteoporosis diet is most effective when tailored to your diagnosis, preferences, lifestyle, and medication regimen. Use these FAQs as a guide for practical nutrition decisions and ongoing adjustments for lifelong bone strength.

# References and Helpful Links

Shen, Y., Huang, X., Wu, J. et al.. The Global Burden of Osteoporosis, Low Bone Mass, and Its Related Fracture in 204 Countries and Territories, 1990-2019. Frontiers in Endocrinology. 2022. doi:10.3389/fendo.2022.882241

Gregson, C., Armstrong, D., Bowden, J. et al.. UK clinical guideline for the prevention and treatment of osteoporosis. Archives of Osteoporosis. 2022. doi:10.1007/s11657-022-01061-5

Kanis, J., Kanis, J.. Assessment of fracture risk and its application to screening for postmenopausal osteoporosis: Synopsis of a WHO report. Osteoporosis International. 1994. doi:10.1007/bf01622200

Gallagher, J. Advances in osteoporosis from to Menopause. doi:10./gme. 19. Accessed February 11, 2026. https://scholar.google.com/citations?user=BSNZxRwAAAAJ&hl=en&oi=sra

Kanis, J., Odén, A., Johansson, H. et al.. Fracture Risk Assessment. https://doi.org/10.1016/b978-0-12-415853-5.00068-6

Curry, S., Krist, A. et al.. Screening for Osteoporosis to Prevent Fractures. https://doi.org/10.1001/jama.2018.7498

Bauer, J., Biolo, G., Cederholm, T. et al.. Evidence-Based Recommendations for Optimal Dietary Protein Intake in Older People: A

Position Paper From the PROT-AGE Study Group. https://doi.org/10.1016/j.jamda.2013.05.021

Holick, M. F. (2007). Vitamin D deficiency. New England journal of medicine, 357(3), 266-281.https://www.nejm.org/doi/abs/10.1056/NEJMra070553

Tucker, K. L., Morita, K., Qiao, N., Hannan, M. T., Cupples, L. A., & Kiel, D. P. (2006). Colas, but not other carbonated beverages, are associated with low bone mineral density in older women: The Framingham Osteoporosis Study. The American journal of clinical nutrition, 84(4), 936-942.https://www.sciencedirect.com/science/article/pii/S0002916523291170

www.ingramcontent.com/pod-product-compliance
Lightning Source LLC
LaVergne TN
LVHW020235210926
848481LV00016B/2218
* 9 7 9 8 2 9 5 7 3 4 4 9 6 *